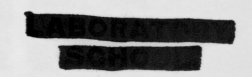

A Finding-Out Book

# THE SENSES

### Seeing, Hearing, Smelling, Tasting, Touching

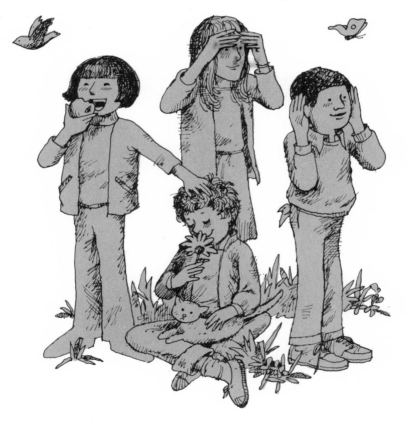

by **John M. Scott**

illustrated by **John E. Johnson**

*Parents' Magazine Press • New York*

Library of Congress Cataloging in Publication Data

Scott, John Martin, 1913-
    The senses—seeing, hearing, smelling, tasting,
touching.

    (A Finding-out book)
    Includes index.
    SUMMARY: Explains the physiology of each of our
five senses.
    1. Senses and sensation—Juvenile literature.
[1. Senses and sensation]    I. Johnson, John Emil,
1929-ill.    II. Title
QP434.S37        612'.8        75-2189
ISBN 0-8193-0821-8

# Contents

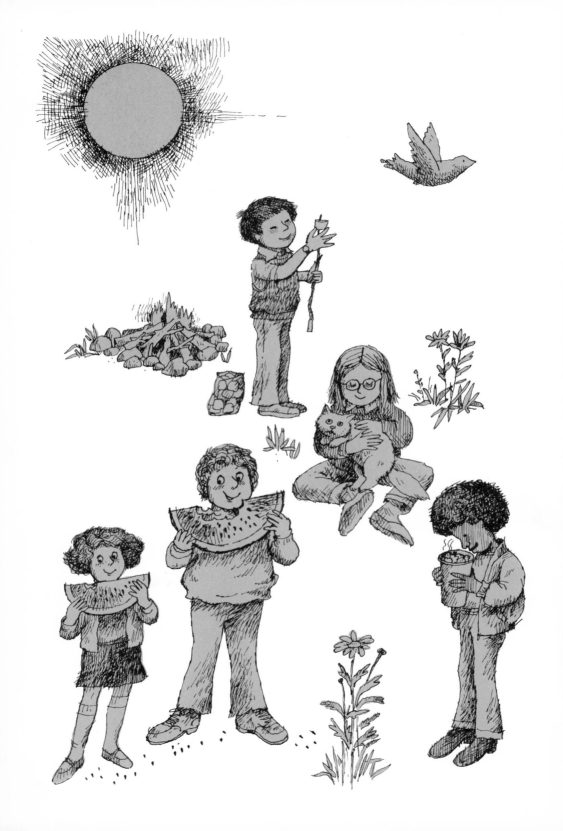

# ONE

# Our Senses

Did you ever stop to think what it would be like if you were born without the gifts of sight, hearing, touch, taste, and smell?

Without sight you would never see the faces of your friends. If you tried to walk you might fall down stairs, stumble over a bench, or bump into a wall. You would live in a world of blackness like a night without end.

Without hearing you would never hear the sound of your name. Your world of blackness would also be a silent world.

Without the other three senses, you would never know the smell of freshly buttered hot popcorn, or the taste of ice cold watermelon. You would never feel the softness of a marshmallow or a cat's fur.

You are somewhat like a king who lives shut up behind the stone walls of his castle and has to depend on messengers to bring him news about the great, wide world that stretches beyond his castle walls.

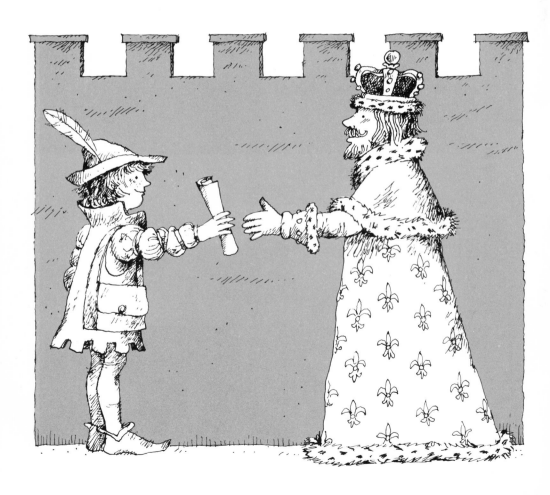

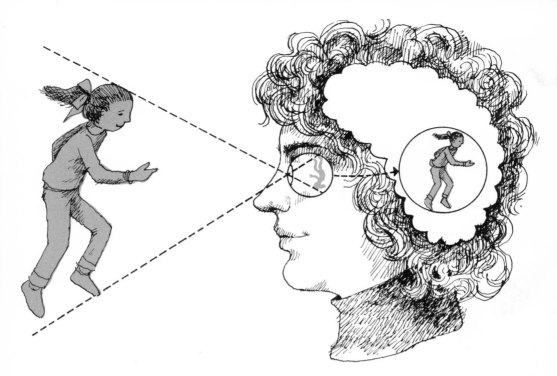

**The eye is a messenger that brings us information.**

Your brain is locked up in silent darkness behind the bony walls of your skull and has to depend on the five senses to bring information about the great wide world that surrounds you.

Centuries ago a very wise man named Aristotle said: "Nothing is in the brain unless it has first been in the senses." Only through our senses—seeing, hearing, smelling, touching, and tasting—do we gain knowledge of ourselves and the world around us.

7

# TWO

# The Gift of Sight

The most important of our senses is sight. Try this. Close your eyes and then, very slowly and carefully, try to walk across the room. If you are like most people, you will feel uneasy with your eyes shut. In a few minutes you will feel such a great need to see that you can no longer keep your eyes shut. You open your eyes with a rush of joy to find yourself once again in contact with the things around you.

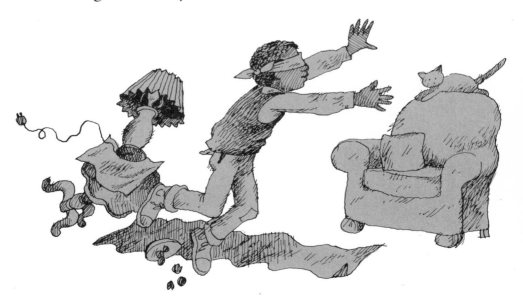

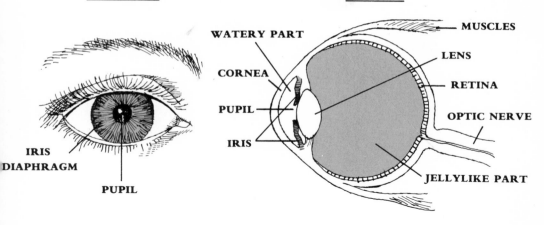

If you look sideways into a mirror, perhaps you may notice a clear, plastic-like covering that bends, or bulges out, at the front part of your eyeball. This clear tissue is called the *cornea*. The cornea is like a tiny glass window on the outside part of your eye. Because the cornea is curved like a half-circle, it helps to bend beams of light. A healthy cornea is one of the clearest tissues in the body.

Look into the eyes of a friend. Perhaps her eyes are brown, blue, or hazel. That circle of color you are looking at is the *iris*. Its job is like that of a shade on a window—to control the amount of light that comes into the eye.

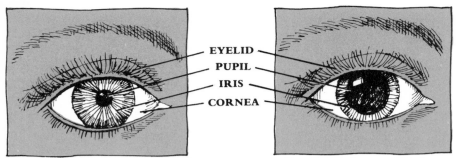

EYELID
PUPIL
IRIS
CORNEA

**In bright light the pupil is smaller.**     **In dim light the pupil is larger.**

In the center of the iris is a round black spot called the pupil. It is really not a separate part, but is the opening in the iris through which the light passes.

The pupil seems to be black because it leads into the inside of the eye. In much the same way, the window of a distant building, even though clear, sometimes appears black in bright sunlight.

We mentioned that the iris might be thought of as a shade on a window. But it does much more. It is also an automatic light meter that measures the amount of light falling on it, and then opens or closes the pupil to let just the right amount of light enter into the eye. On a bright day the iris makes the pupil very small. On a cloudy day, or in the evening, the iris makes the pupil much bigger.

To show how fast the iris can change its size
to control the amount of light entering the eye,
try this experiment. In the evening stand by a
bright lamp. Use a hand mirror to see how small
the iris is. Now walk into a dimly lit corner of
the room. Again look into the mirror and see
what has happened to the iris.

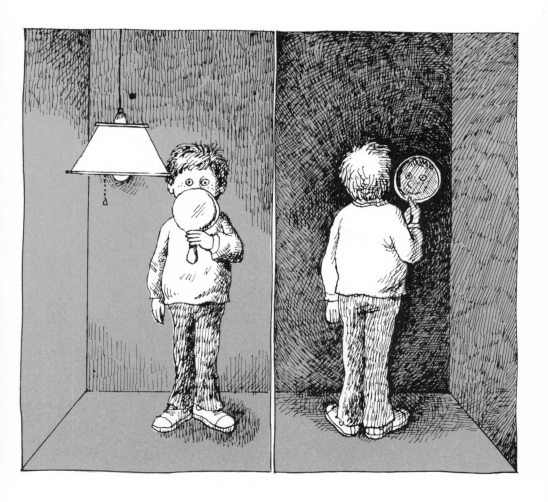

Before you take a picture with an expensive camera you must adjust the *diaphragm* (*dye*-uh-fram) or opening in front of the lens to admit the proper amount of light. The iris of your eye is a combination light meter and self-adjusting diaphragm.

When you walk from a darkened room into bright sunlight, the iris expands to cover more of the pupil, making the pupil smaller. In the evening, the iris contracts, or grows smaller, increasing the size of the pupil to let in more light.

Behind the pupil of your eye is the *lens.* Its purpose is the same as the lens in a camera—to make a clear, sharp picture or image, to bring things into focus. When we say a thing is in focus, we mean that its image or picture inside the eye—or inside a camera—is sharp and clear. There are, however, some big differences between the lens in a camera and the lens in your eye.

The lens in a camera is a solid piece of glass made into a convex or bulging shape. The lens

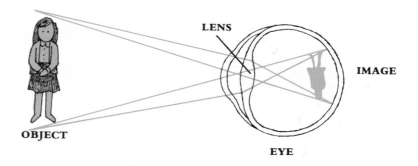

LENS

IMAGE

OBJECT

EYE

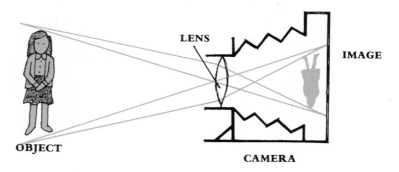

LENS

IMAGE

OBJECT

CAMERA

**The iris of the eye is like the light meter in a camera. Both measure the amount of light and adjust the opening.**

in a camera may be moved forward or backward until a clear, sharp picture or image is made on the film.

The lens in your eye is soft, like Jello or jelly. It is held in place by a broad sheet of material that reminds you of a sheet of plastic. Unlike the

13

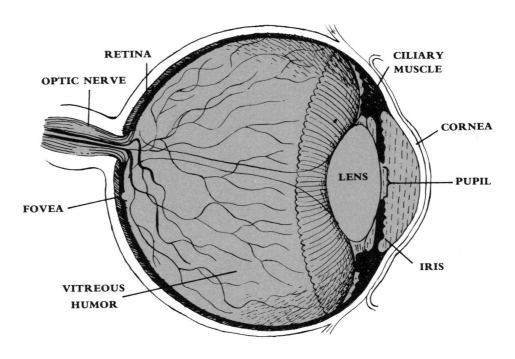

lens in a camera, the lens in the eye does not move forward or backward to get a clear picture. It changes its shape. This change in the shape of the lens of the eye is brought about by the pull of a ring of muscle called the *ciliary* (*sill*-ee-airy) muscle, which is attached to the sheet that holds the lens in place.

If you have normal vision, you can look at a nearby object, such as this book, and then at a distant object, such as a tall building six blocks away, and both will be in focus.

Eye muscles act very fast to change the shape
of the lens in your eye so that you always have
a clear view of the world around you. As you read
this page, the lens must be thick to focus the print
on to the *retina* (*rett*-tin-uh), the back part of
your eye. When you watch a high-flying
wedge-shaped band of geese honking their way
south in the autumn sky, the lens becomes thin.
When you look at distant objects the muscles
around the lens are relaxed, or at rest.

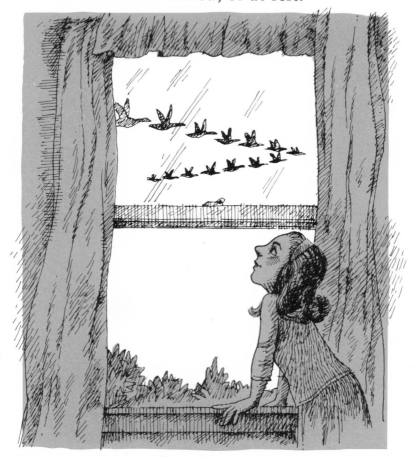

If you read for a long time or do other kinds of close work, the muscles become tired. Be kind to your eyes and rest them now and then by looking at distant objects or by closing them for a short time.

Some people can see things that are far away more clearly than nearby objects. In these farsighted people the distance between the lens and the retina is too short, or the lens may be so flat that it does not bend the light beams enough.

Farsightedness can be corrected with convex lenses. Convex is a Latin word that means curved

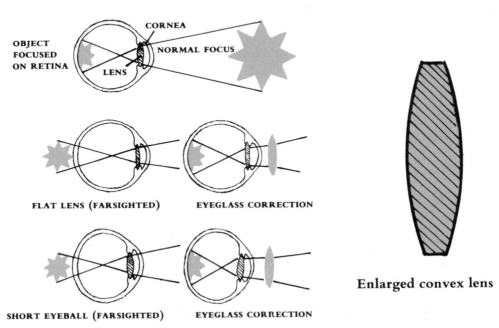

OBJECT FOCUSED ON RETINA

CORNEA

NORMAL FOCUS

LENS

FLAT LENS (FARSIGHTED)

EYEGLASS CORRECTION

SHORT EYEBALL (FARSIGHTED)

EYEGLASS CORRECTION

Enlarged convex lens

or rounded. A convex lens is rounded like the outside of a ping pong ball. It is thicker in the middle than at the edge. The curved surface of the lens pulls the light rays together so that the images of nearby objects are focused on the retina.

Since the rays of beams of light passing through a convex lens are bent inward and come together in a cone of light, a convex lens is also called a converging lens. It brings the rays of light closer together.

Some people can easily see things that are near to them, but can't see distant objects. In these nearsighted people the eyeball is too long, or the lens is so thick that light rays from distant objects come together or converge to make an image in front of the retina instead of on it.

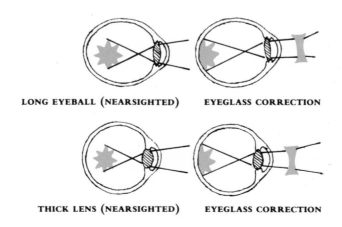

LONG EYEBALL (NEARSIGHTED)     EYEGLASS CORRECTION

THICK LENS (NEARSIGHTED)     EYEGLASS CORRECTION

How can we make the image move back onto the retina?

Nearsightedness can be corrected with concave lenses. Concave is a Latin word that means curved in. A concave lens curves inward like the bowl of a spoon. It is thinner in the center than it is at the edge. This caved-in lens scatters, or throws apart, the beams of light that go through it. A concave lens is a diverging lens that pushes the beams of light apart.

When a person wears concave lenses, the curved-in surface spreads apart the light rays before they enter the eye. As a result of this spreading out of the rays of light, the image is formed at a greater distance from the lens of the eye, and is brought to focus on the retina.

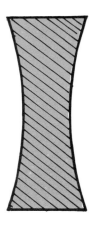 **Enlarged concave lens**

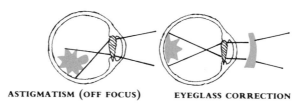

**ASTIGMATISM (OFF FOCUS)**      **EYEGLASS CORRECTION**

Besides nearsightedness and farsightedness there is another defect of the eye called *astigmatism*. It is the failure of the eye to see different parts of an object distinctly at the same time.

Because of its curved shape the cornea acts as a converging lens. If the surface of the cornea does not have the same amount of curve in all places, light rays will be bent more in one part of it than in another. A blurred, fuzzy image is thrown on the retina. Unequal curvature of the surface of the cornea causes astigmatism. Special glass lenses are used to correct astigmatism.

**Look at this wheel with one eye at a time. If you have astigmatism, some of the spokes in the wheel will be clear and in focus while others will be less clear and out of focus.**

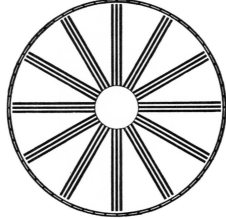

The space back of the lens in the eyeball is filled with a clear, jellylike material through which the light passes on its way to the retina. This clear, colorless material is called the *vitreous humor*. Vitreous is a Latin word meaning glass-like. Humor is a Latin word meaning fluid.

When you are taking pictures with an ordinary camera, you must keep it supplied with fresh film. After the film is exposed, it must be developed and printed before you have a picture. The brain interprets the image on the retina as an erect picture in an instant. As you let your eyes travel around the room, the retina responds to one image after another. You never have to replace any film. New images are formed as old ones fade away. The retina in the eye is like the film in a camera, but it is far better than any man-made film.

The retina is a living tissue of about 130 million cells, sensitive to light. When light hits them, they go to work. There are two kinds of cells— *rods* and *cones*, so named because of their shape.

Cones work in daylight and give us color vision. Rods give us only black and white. Cones are most numerous at the *fovea,* a very small pit, or tiny spot, in the retina, where the eye gets its sharpest images.

The rods and cones are connected to the *optic nerve.* The optic nerve may be compared to a telegraph cable that gives the brain a private line to what is going on in your world. The place where the optic nerve enters the retina is called the blind spot. Any image formed on this spot cannot be seen.

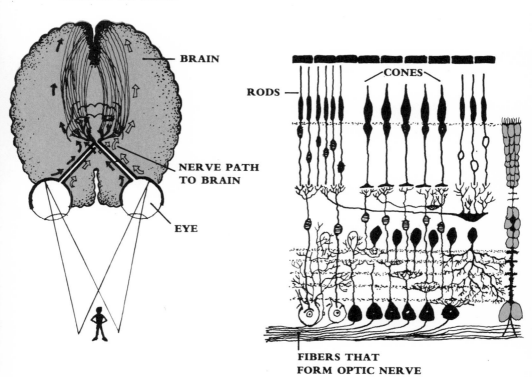

BRAIN

RODS

CONES

NERVE PATH
TO BRAIN

EYE

FIBERS THAT
FORM OPTIC NERVE

To experiment with the blind spot, try this:

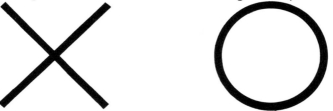

Hold this page about 20 inches away from your eyes, close your left eye, and look at the letter X with your right eye. You will still see the letter O in the corner of your eye. Now slowly bring the book closer to your eyes. At a certain distance, the letter O will vanish.

This is the position where the image falls on the blind spot—the place where the nerves of the retina come together and go to the brain through the optic nerve.

Oddly enough the brain itself never directly experiences the form of energy we call light. The brain rests in darkness inside your skull.

Your eyes change the energy of light into electrical signals that are sent along the optic nerve to the brain. When this electricity reaches your brain, your brain interprets, or translates, these electrical signals into what we call sight.

Sometimes when the signals are not entirely clear, the brain makes a mistake in translating or decoding. Then our eyes may fool us. This is because only part of what we see comes through the eyes; much comes from the mind—past

Stare at the black and white diagram shown above. Do you see gray dots in the white lines where the black squares meet? If you do, look at just one of them. Do you still see them?

experiences, imaginings, desires, and other things that make illusions and often fill in parts of a picture not really there.

When we are fooled by our eyes, it is not because light bouncing off an object did not reach the retina. It is because the brain got its signals mixed up. *Optical illusions* show that seeing is not always believing.

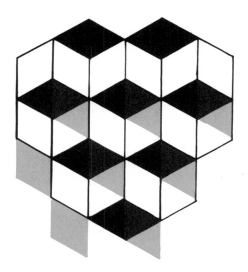

**How many cubes do you count? Turn the picture upside down and count again.**

**Which horizontal line is longest? Measure them.**

**Does this book fold in or out?**

**Which line is longer—AB or BC? Measure them.**

**Which of the three black poles is the tallest? Measure them.**

Even though we think we see people running, walking, and jumping in motion pictures, the truth is that the pictures are not moving pictures. If you look at a motion picture film you will find that each picture is still. The people are not moving around on the film. Why, then, do we think we see people moving when the film is shown on a screen? Because of *persistence of vision*.

As new images are formed on the retina of your eye, the old ones fade away. They don't vanish at once, however. The time needed for an image to disappear is about one-tenth of a second.

Did you ever light a 4th of July sparkler and whirl it in a circle on a dark night? You thought you were looking at a circle of fire! Yet you knew you had only one sparkler, and the fire could be at only one spot at one time.

The same persistence of vision that accounts for the continuous bright circle when you whirled the sparkler also accounts for the illusion of continuous motion when you see a movie. When you watch a motion picture you are watching a

series of separate still pictures that are flashed on
the screen at the rate of about 24 pictures in one
second, with a short period of darkness between
each picture.

Here is how it works. The motion picture
projector throws one stationary, or still, picture on
the screen for about one-thirtieth of a second.
Then a shutter comes down in front of the lens
of the projector and cuts off the light. During this
time, when the room is in darkness, the film is
moved down so that the next picture is in place.
Now the shutter opens, and the next still picture
is flashed on the screen. Because your eye keeps
an image on the retina longer than it actually is
there and blends it with the next image, you think
you see motion.

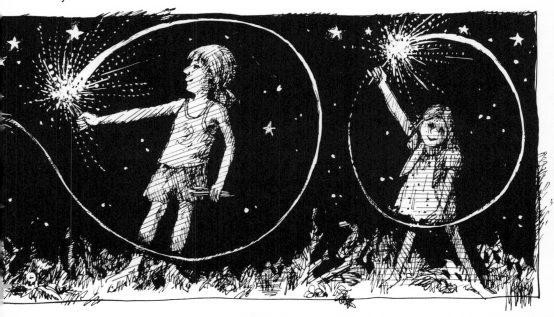

To show a boy raising his arm, for example, each one of the series of pictures would show the arm in slightly higher position. In the time that such an action might take, say one second, 24 pictures will be thrown on the screen. You are not aware of the individual pictures. All blend together to give the illusion of motion on the screen. Television also depends on persistence of vision.

Did you ever turn on a TV set and find that you could get the picture but no sound? Pictures without sound give us some idea of how our life would be if we could see things but could not hear what was going on around us. Next to the gift of sight, the most important sense is that of hearing, which we will talk about next.

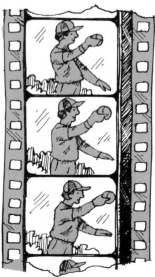

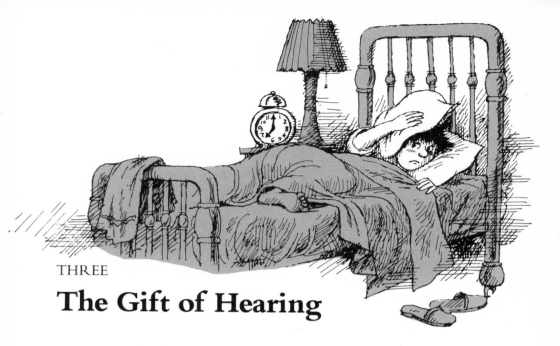

# THREE

# The Gift of Hearing

Can you find out what is happening without looking?

The answer is "Yes." Even though you are not looking, you can tell when someone behind you pops a balloon, crumples a newspaper, blows a whistle, toots a horn, or uses a pencil sharpener.

One big difference between our eyes and our ears is that we can close our eyes and shut out the world of light. We can't close our ears. Since our ears are always open, we can use an alarm clock to pull us out of dreamland. Our eyes can't see the hands of the clock in the dark, but our ears tell us that it is time to get up.

29

When the gong hits the bell on the alarm clock, the metal vibrates, or moves back and forth. Vibrating objects are the source of sound. The bell pushes against the air and sets tiny particles of air into motion. This motion or vibration of the air is what we call sound. The moving particles of air hit your eardrum and make it vibrate.

As we will see, these vibrations are brought to our inner ears, where nerves change the sound vibrations into electrical signals which are sent to the brain.

If you blow a dog whistle, you probably won't hear it. Blow the whistle when a dog is near and watch what happens. Some animals can hear sounds that humans cannot. The human ear can hear only those things that vibrate from about 20 to 20,000 times a second.

If you turn up the volume on your radio you can do more than hear it. Touch the cabinet with your fingers, and you will feel it vibrate.

The fleshy outer part of your ear, called the

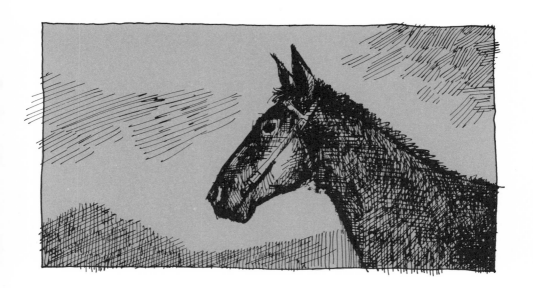

*pinna*, has the job of collecting sounds and leading them into the opening that goes to the middle ear.

The next time you see a horse, notice its ears. The pinnae of horses' ears not only stand up tall and wide, but they can be turned to listen to sounds coming from different directions.

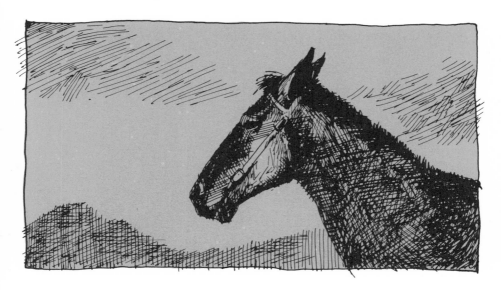

You can increase the collecting power of your pinnae by pushing them forward and cupping them with your hands. Even better, get a megaphone and hold the small end over your ear. (You can make your own megaphone by rolling a newspaper into a cone shape. Put the small end of the cone next to your ear and listen.)

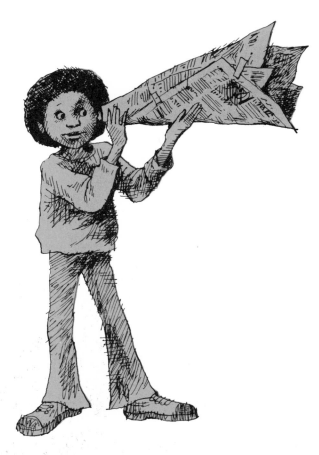

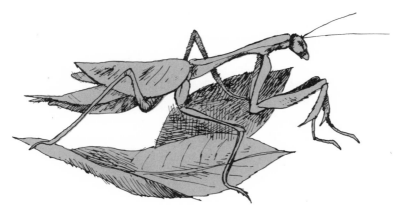

Our ears, of course, are on our heads, and so are the ears of cats, dogs, and other animals. But that interesting insect, the praying mantis, has ears on its front legs. And snakes do not have ears at all. They feel vibrations through their bodies. The outer ear of a goldfish looks like two lines along the side of its body. Goldfish are very sensitive to vibrations. That is why you should not tap on the glass of the goldfish bowl.

**You can't see them, but the ears of a goldfish are like two lines on the side of its body.**

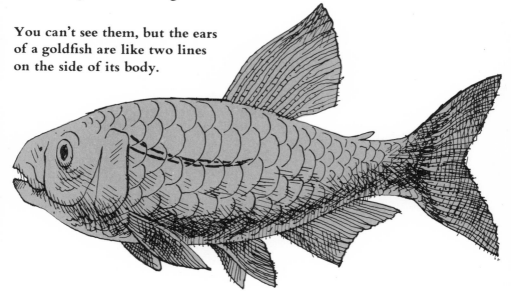

The eardrum is just that—a tiny, drum-like skin, or sensitive *membrane* that separates the outer ear from the middle ear. Sound waves striking the eardrum cause it to move or vibrate. The eardrum sets into motion three small bones (the *ossicles*)

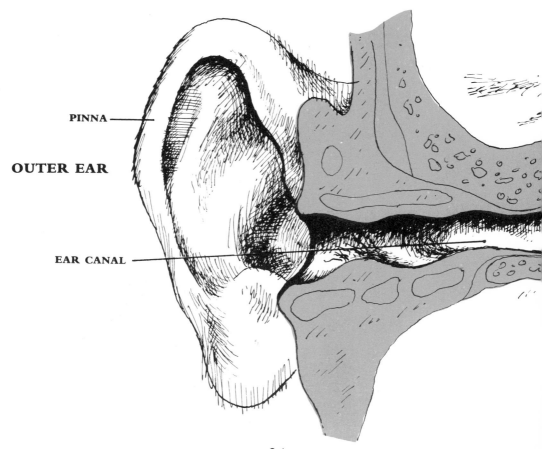

PINNA

OUTER EAR

EAR CANAL

in the middle ear. These are the *hammer,* the *anvil,* and the *stirrup,* the three smallest bones in the body. Extending from the inner surface of the eardrum to another membrane that covers the opening between the middle ear and the inner ear, the three bones form a bridge across the middle ear.

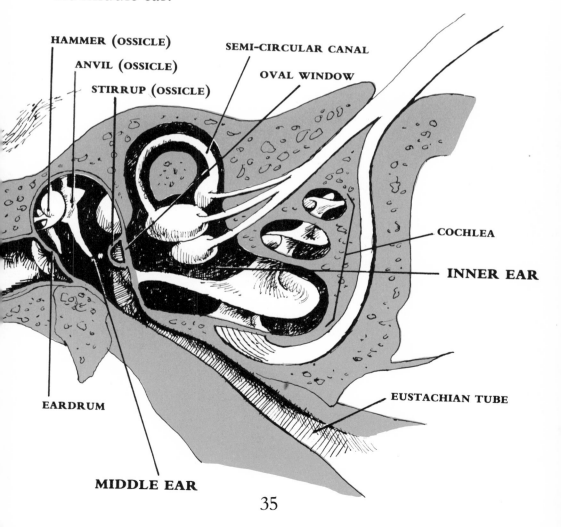

HAMMER (OSSICLE)

ANVIL (OSSICLE)

STIRRUP (OSSICLE)

SEMI-CIRCULAR CANAL

OVAL WINDOW

COCHLEA

INNER EAR

EARDRUM

EUSTACHIAN TUBE

MIDDLE EAR

Inside the inner ear is a somewhat snail-shaped tube, the *cochlea* (*cock*-lee-uh). It contains a fluid and the tiny hairlike endings of the nerve that brings messages to the brain. As the stirrup vibrates against the membrane covering the oval window—the opening between the middle and the inner ear—the vibrations are passed to the fluid in the cochlea. The endings of this nerve change the movements into electrical signs which are sent to the brain. These electrical impulses are interpreted by the brain as sounds.

The eardrum is easily injured. Never try to remove wax or any foreign matter from your ear by using a pencil, toothpick, hairpin, or any sharp, pointed instrument.

You should never shout into a person's ear. A loud sound can make the eardrum vibrate so much it may cause damage. Also, you should never strike anyone on the side of the head. Any sudden change in pressure can injure the eardrum.

If you use ear plugs when you swim, always take them out slowly. If you pull them out like

a cork from a bottle, you make a low pressure
on the outside of the eardrum. The air trapped
on the other side can rush out and break, or
rupture, the eardrum.

Have you noticed a popping or ringing in your
ears when you go up in an elevator, or take off
in an airplane? The ringing is due to the changes
in air pressure on the outside of your eardrum.

You can help make the pressure equal by
opening your mouth, yawning, or chewing gum,
for there is a connection, or opening, between the

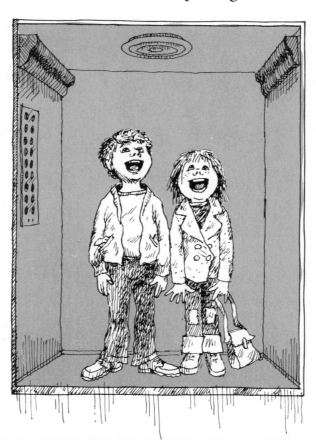

throat and the middle ear known as the *Eustachian* (you-*stay*-she-un) tube. Its purpose is not to help you hear but to equalize the air pressure on both sides of the eardrum.

Soldiers firing big guns open their mouths so that the sudden blast of air on the outside will not push on their eardrums hard enough to injure them.

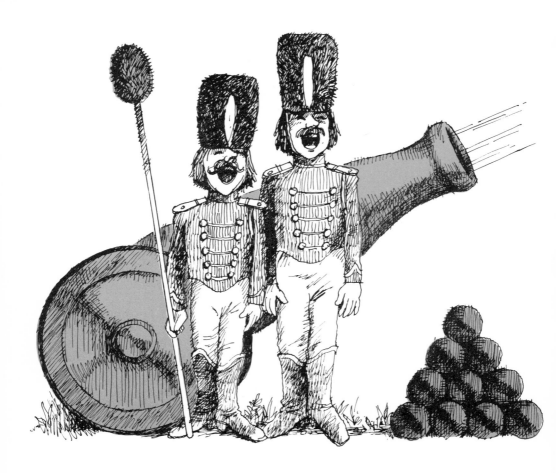

You may have found that you could not hear as well when you had a cold. That is because the Eustachian tube was probably swollen partly shut.

When you blow your nose, remember that there is an air connection between your nose, throat, and ears. If you close your mouth and pinch your nostrils when you blow your nose, air will be forced up the Eustachian tube and against your eardrums. This blast of air against your eardrums could hurt them, and even cause them to rupture, or break.

The inner ear also has a structure which, like the Eustachian tube, has nothing to do with hearing. It is made of three small tubes shaped like semicircles and set together in such a way that they look like a pretzel pulled out of shape. These semicircular canals help you keep your sense of balance. If you have a cold or an ear infection, they may be affected and cause you to get dizzy.

In the United States there are about 100,000 people who cannot hear. They live in a world that

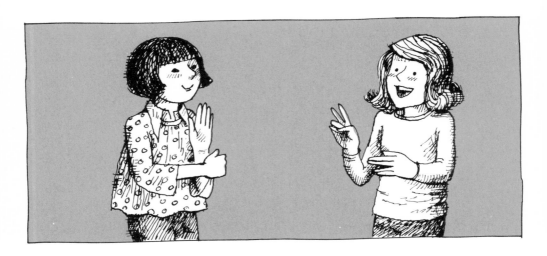

is as silent as the moon. Since many of them have never heard anyone speak, they cannot use their own voices unless they are given special speech lessons.

The deaf are forced to replace their hearing with other senses. Most of them do this by sight, through sign language, and by lip reading. Some deaf people can tell what people are saying by placing their fingers on the speaker's vocal cords.

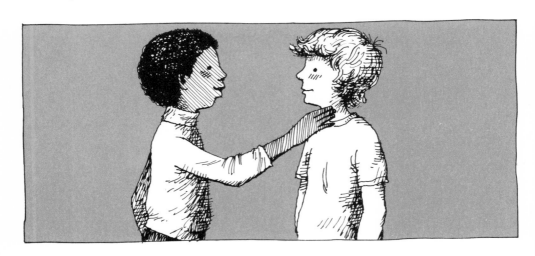

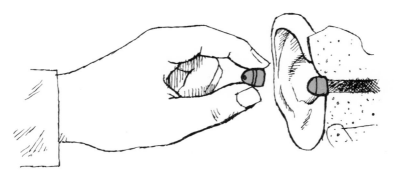

This air-conduction hearing aid goes into the ear. This actual-size photograph shows that the hearing aid is about the size of a man's thumb.

Many people who are deaf or hard of hearing are helped by hearing aids. The hearing aids have a small electrical device which makes the sound louder. In the *air-conduction* hearing aid, the receiver is put into the outer ear and sends increased vibrations to the middle ear. In the *bone-conduction* hearing aid, the receiver is clamped

In the bone-conduction hearing aid the receiver is clamped to the bone behind the ear. Vibrations are sent through the bones of the head into the inner ear.

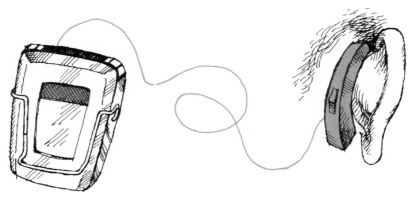

to the bone behind the ear. Vibrations are sent through the bones of the head into the inner ear. Bone carries sound better than air.

Even though you have been talking most of your life, you may never have heard your voice as others hear it. The sound of your own voice comes to you by bone conduction, while others hear you by air conduction.

When you talk, your tongue, vocal cords, and lips move back and forth, and set the air into motion. They do even more. They make the bones in your head rattle and shake. To prove it, place your hand firmly on top of your head; then talk loudly, or sing. You will feel your head shake, or vibrate.

So far in this book we have found out about the senses of sight and hearing. Can you think of a sense that may tell you about things you may not be able to see at the moment and do not hear? It can at times tell you about things in another room, long before you enter the room itself.

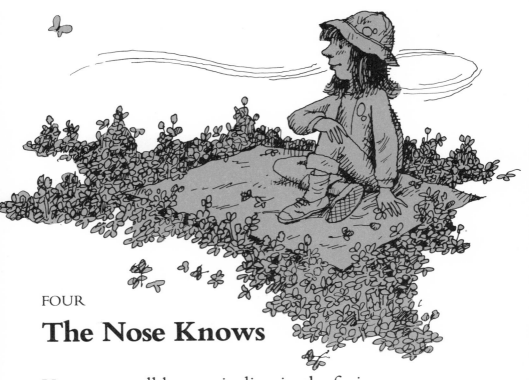

FOUR

# The Nose Knows

You can smell bacon sizzling in the frying pan, moth balls in your closet, or freshly cut clover in June because tiny particles, or bits of matter called *molecules,* jump up from these different things, then race through the air to punch you in the nose!

In the upper part of each nostril there is a flat membrane or piece of skin about the size of a postage stamp. Sticking out of the membrane, like so many lines on a telephone switchboard, are tiny hairs. When an odor reaches these hairs, they send an electrical signal or impulse racing along nerves that lead to your brain. Your brain translates or interprets these electrical signals as smells.

Like your sense of hearing, your nose can operate in the dark. If you are walking through the woods at night, your sense of smell may tell you that a skunk has been around, even though you don't see it.

Your sense of smell brings you information without the use of words. If someone in the house has washed her hair with a perfumed shampoo, you know it without being told. If someone is cooking with garlic, you know it the moment you enter the kitchen!

What accounts for our attraction to pleasant smells? Science does not fully understand the *olfactory* organ, or sense of smell. Your nose can receive and sort out odors with a speed and exactness that no scientific instrument or machine can equal.

You notice that a young woman is wearing perfume as sweet as apple blossoms. You may be smelling an amount of perfume so small that no machine known could either find it, or tell what it is. Scientists believe that the human nose can pick out as little as one-trillionth of an ounce of a strong-smelling chemical.

As far as we know now, there may be no limit to the number of smells the human nose can recognize or pick out.

Although our skill at picking out odors is good, some animals have an even better sense of smell. If the wind is right, a deer can smell a person more than one hundred yards away.

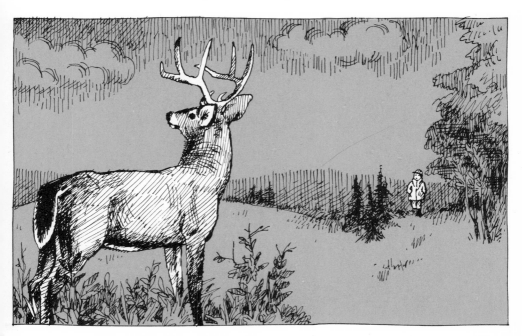

It has been said that the nose, not the tongue, really enjoys food. Much of what people call tasting is really smelling. If you have a head cold, and your nose is stuffed up, you will have trouble tasting your food.

Some afternoon you may wish to invite a few friends to your home for a tasting game. Before they come, cut a slice from an apple into small parts, and put them in a cup. Do the same with a slice of potato.

When your friends arrive, blindfold them. While your blindfolded friends hold their noses shut, place a small piece of apple on each one's tongue. Ask them to tell you what it is. Then do the same with a small piece of potato.

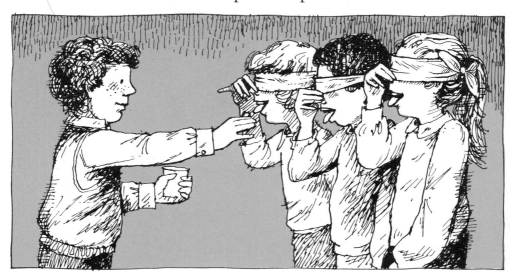

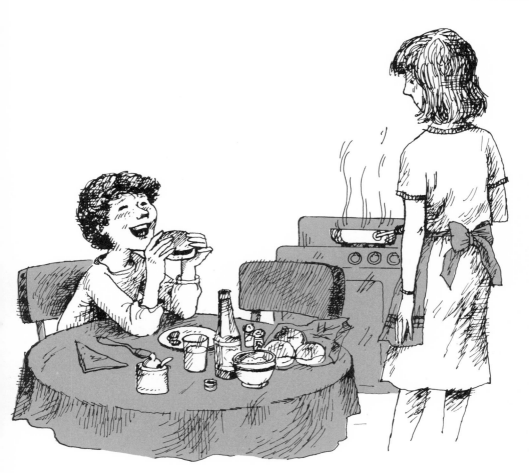

Can your friends tell you what the foods are when their noses are blocked so they cannot smell them?

When the delightful aroma from a sizzling hamburger drifts into your nostrils, the work of your nose is only beginning. Not until you have put the meat into your mouth does smell come into full play. As you chew, you free odors that rise through the back of your mouth into the inner parts of your nose, where the olfactory nerve is located. It is there that you discover the delights of meat that is done to a turn, or enjoy the tingling tang of a Coke.

Our sense of smell can act as a lifeguard to warn us of gasoline fumes in the air, or gas escaping from a leaky pipe in the basement. The smell of smoke—long before the smoke was seen—has warned families of hidden fires in attics.

Special aromas are like index cards to memory banks in our mind. Our sense of smell is tied to our past. Some aromas stir up memories so strong that we relive the past. Suppose you could smell separately—at different times—such things as peppermint, cinnamon, vanilla, chocolate, camphor, or rain on a dusty road? What would they make you think of that happened to you some time ago?

And now can you think of the sense you have that goes to work only when you put something into your mouth?

# FIVE

# The Taste Tells

Thanks to your taste buds, each meal can bring delight to your day. Your tongue has three thousand taste buds, each with its nerve connection to the brain. No one knows exactly how these taste buds work. Some scientists think that particles of food fit into them like light plugs into sockets, closing circuits and sending electrical impulses to the brain. The brain interprets the signals to mean: "The strawberry ice cream is delicious." "The lemon is sour." "The potatoes need salt."

Scientists know that the senses of taste and smell differ in one important way from the senses of sight, hearing, and touch. They are both chemical senses. Things that give us taste must come into direct contact with taste buds. These are on our tongues. Taste buds on the tip of your tongue are most responsive to sweet. Those further back respond to salty, sour, and bitter tastes.

If you would like to find out what parts of your tongue are sensitive to different tastes, take a toothpick and put a drop of salt water on different parts of your tongue. What parts are most sensitive to salt?

Take a fresh toothpick and repeat the experiment with sugar water; then try lemon juice and bitter chocolate.

The tongue is something like a small chemistry laboratory with different taste buds to inform us of the sweetness of honey, the sour taste of dill pickles, and the salty taste of cod fish.

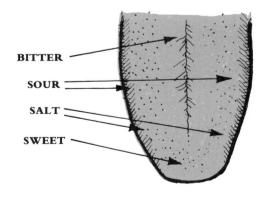

TONGUE

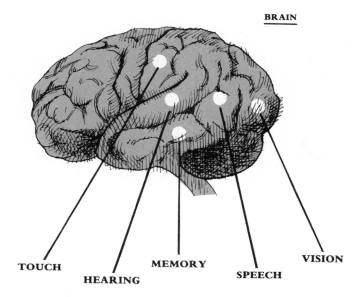

**BRAIN**

TOUCH          MEMORY               VISION
      HEARING              SPEECH

Besides tasting, the tongue helps you eat by forcing food against your teeth. Then it helps in swallowing the food.

Your tongue also helps you talk. To prove how necessary your tongue is for speaking, try keeping your tongue flat on the floor of your mouth and pronouncing such words as *snap, clack, teeth,* and *splash.*

So far we have found out about our senses of sight, hearing, smell, and taste. There is still the fifth sense that tells us about things only if we make contact with objects around us and touch them.

51

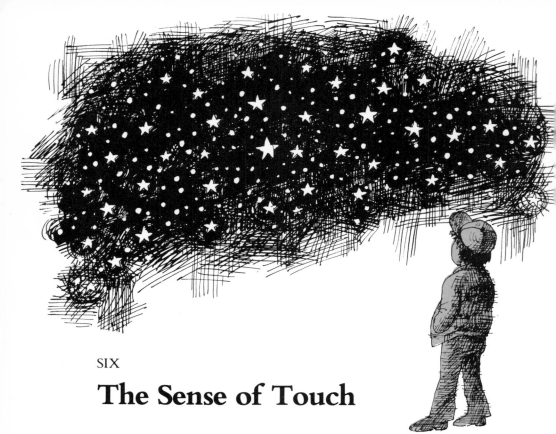

SIX

# The Sense of Touch

Touch is the sense that puts us in the most direct contact with the world around us. Our eyes can see stars sparkling on the far side of the Milky Way galaxy. Our ears can hear the distant roar of a waterfall. Our nose can smell bacon frying. Our taste buds tell us about things that are mixed with the moisture on our tongue. But the sense of touch depends on direct contact. Touch gives us a sense of love that no other sense can supply.

According to scientists, love comes most of all from close bodily contact in the early months of life. Babies who are not given human contact, who are not hugged and picked up, die just as surely as if they had been starved.

We are not satisfied to simply look at the things we like. We want to touch them, to embrace them, to hold them close to our hearts.

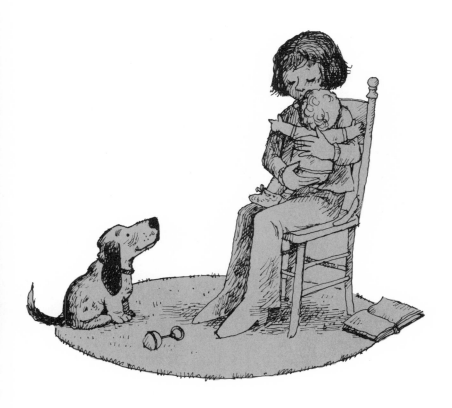

The sensation of touch can help tell what things are without looking. To prove it, get a big paper bag like those used in supermarkets. Into the bag put such things as a ping pong ball, a marble, a rock, a piece of sandpaper, a piece of silk, and some nails. If you can't find those particular things, any assortment of things of different shapes and textures will do. Blindfold a friend and ask him or her to reach into the bag and pull out one thing at a time, telling you what it is. How many times did you get the right answer?

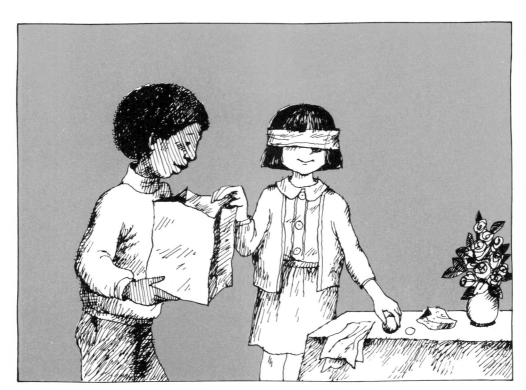

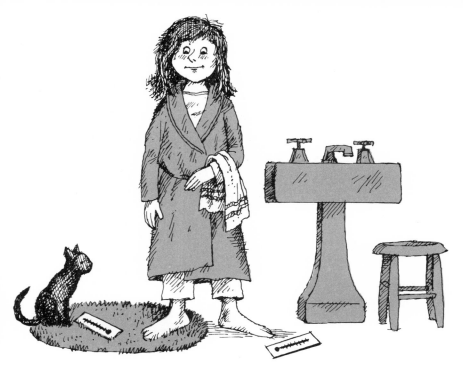

Sometimes our sense of touch can fool us. On a cold winter morning stand in the bathroom with one bare foot touching the tile floor and the other bare foot on a rug. The rug and the tile are the same temperature. (You can prove that by putting thermometers on both the floor and the rug.) Yet the tile floor seems colder!

The reason for this is that the tile is a good conductor, which means that it takes the heat away from your foot very rapidly. The rug, on the other hand, is a poor conductor, and does not take the heat away from your foot as rapidly.

The nerve endings most sensitive to pressure are close together in the tips of the fingers, the bottom of the thumb, the palm, and the lips. The tip of your nose is also sensitive, as you know when you tickle it with a feather.

On your arm and back the nerve endings that report pressure are much farther apart. Try this experiment: keep your eyes closed, or wear a blindfold while a friend touches the points of two pencils at different spots on your back.

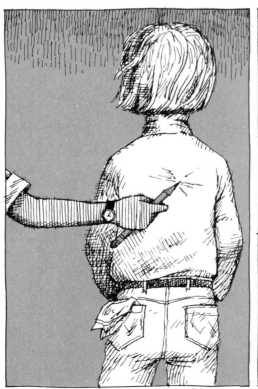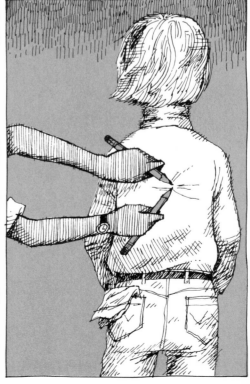

Without telling you how many pencils he is using, your friend will touch your skin with only one pencil at times. At other times the friend will use both pencils, keeping their points about one-quarter of an inch apart. Can you tell him when he is using one or two pencils?

Now let your friend keep increasing the distance between the pencils when he touches your skin with their points. How far apart do the pencils have to be before you feel them as two points?

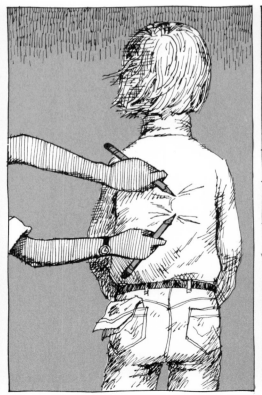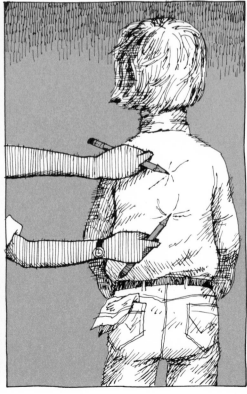

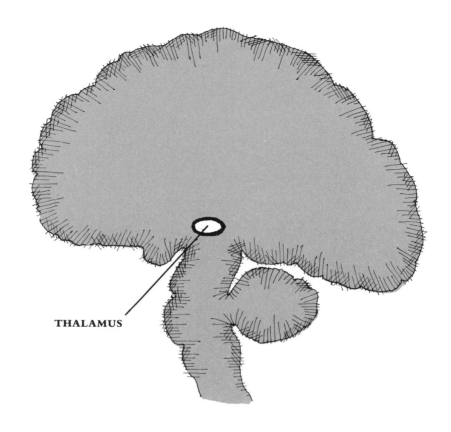

**THALAMUS**

Although much about the sensation of pain is still unknown, scientists have found that pain is a coded electrical signal of impulse sent to the brain from different parts of your body. The part of your brain called the *thalamus* (*thal*-uh-muss) interprets these signals as pain.

Let's see what happens if you stub your big toe.

First, there are nerve endings in the skin called *receptors*. These nerve endings change the energy of impact, when your toe hits something hard, into a code of electrical nerve impulses. The nerve impulses are then sent by nerve fibers from the toe to the spinal cord. Some electrical messages race up your spinal cord at speeds up to 300 miles an hour. Your brain translates, or interprets, these electrical signals as pain.

**This network can carry up to three million messages in a second.**

Strange as it may seem, some people are born without the sense of pain. They can be stuck with pins and plunge their feet into ice cold water or steam and feel no pain.

This may sound wonderful, but it is really quite dangerous. Imagine placing your hand on a hot stove and not knowing that your flesh is burning.

A pain-free boy wondered why he could not jump over a tennis net. He was found to have a broken thigh bone.

A pain-free girl broke her ankle, but didn't know it until the ankle swelled so much she couldn't put her shoe on.

Taste and smell, as we have seen, are chemical senses. Like hearing, touch is a mechanical, or impact, sense. Before a nerve ending

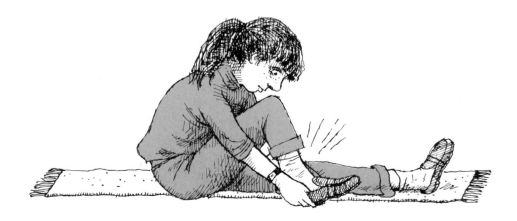

can send an electric signal or message to your brain, something must move the sensory nerve.

If someone jabs you in the ribs, the first feeling takes place when the sensory nerves near the surface of the skin send signals to your brain that something has made contact.

These sensory nerves or touch receptors are not evenly distributed over your body. A spot on the end of your fingertip or tongue, not bigger than the end of the eraser on your pencil, may have over 100 receptors. A spot the same size on the back of your hand may have only ten.

Where there are hairs on your body, nerves wrapped around their bases seem to give you pressure feelings. In some hairless parts of the body, pressure seems to be felt on the skin by means of free nerve endings—fine, naked threads of nerves.

The touch of another person can often say what cannot be put in words. A gentle hug, a warm embrace, a tender kiss, a pat on the back, a head on the shoulder, holding hands—all these are touching ways to say "I love you."

How wonderful the sense of touch! It lets us explore the shape of a tulip's cup, and the small, cool grape. It brings us the delight of summer sun, and, best of all, it gives us the warmth of friendship when hand meets hand.

How wonderful all our senses are! Our eyes tell us the shape, color, and size of things. Our ears tell us what sounds things are making. Our sense of smell gives us their aroma. Our sense of taste tells us whether things are sweet, salty, sour, or bitter. Our sense of touch tells us whether things are smooth, rough, hot, cold, dry, wet, slippery, bumpy, soft, or hard. Altogether our senses make our lives interesting and exciting.

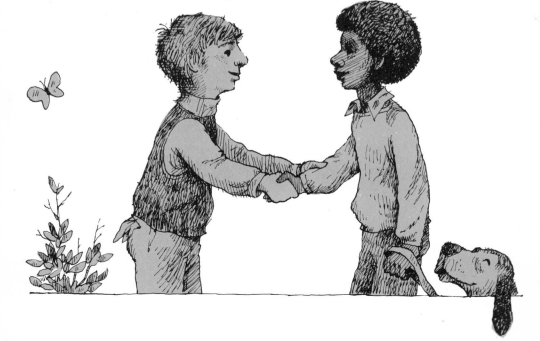

# Index